CAREERS IN
NEUROLOGY
NEUROSCIENCE

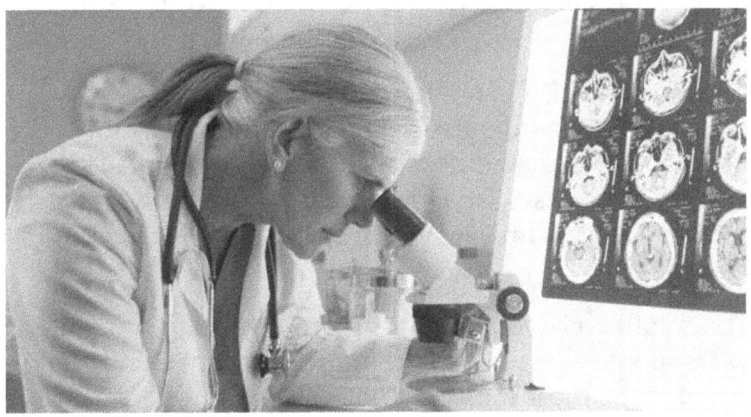

NEUROLOGY IS A MEDICAL SPECIALTY that deals with disorders of the nervous system, which includes the brain, spinal cord, and nerves. Because the brain acts as the control center for the entire body, neural problems may affect body parts. For example, multiple sclerosis can affect numerous parts of the body including eyes, skin, and leg or arm muscles. Neurology is such a vast field that most neurologists devote their practice to a particular subspecialty like pediatrics, head trauma, brain cancer, or seizure disorders such as epilepsy, or speech disorders. Neurosurgery is also a subspecialty. Neurosurgeons, commonly known as brain surgeons, operate on the nervous system, but typically do not follow up with long-term care.

Neurology is considered a frontier field of medicine. There is much more to be learned about the human brain and that is where neuroscientists come in. Neuroscientists research anything related to the nervous system to learn more about how it works and what causes neurological disorders. It is a scientific discipline that is uncovering new secrets of the brain every day. As the neuroscientists discover new ways to diagnose and treat health problems, neurologists are able to offer more hope to the millions of Americans who suffer from nervous system disorders.

Getting into this field requires a long and rigorous education. A neurologist will need to earn a medical degree, whereas a neuroscientist will usually pursue a PhD. In some cases, an individual will have both. In total, it takes 12 years on average to become a fully practicing neurologist.

You might well wonder if it is worth investing so many years of intense study. Neurologists overwhelmingly say yes, it is the most fulfilling and meaningful career imaginable. The work can certainly be demanding and stressful when a life is on the line, but throughout your career, you will see your hard work pay off in numerous ways. The pay is certainly generous, but no one goes into this career for the money. There are more exciting job opportunities than there are candidates, guaranteeing you a variety of options before you even finish your schooling. You get to work with intelligent and highly motivated people who are as committed as you are to making advances in the field of neurology. Most of all, you will get to work on some of the most interesting and complex cases in medicine.

WHAT YOU CAN DO NOW

PREPARATION FOR A CAREER IN NEUROLOGY should start early in high school. A guidance counselor can help create a curriculum that will meet college entrance requirements. In general, that will mean four years each of English, mathematics, and natural sciences. Students who plan to major in college in biological sciences or a pre-med track should perform well in advanced biology, chemistry, and physics courses. Any other classes related to health or psychology will be helpful.

Neurologists need good communications skills to deal with other healthcare professionals and patients that may be of any age or background. A foreign language can also be very useful since neurologists often work with patients who do not speak English. Becoming fluent in a language such as Spanish may help a candidate for medical school stand out. Future neuroscience researchers should take classes that will strengthen their writing skills so they can eventually write papers that will be published.

Get involved in relevant extracurricular activities, especially those that offer leadership opportunities. Joining a science club that involves laboratory work is a good way to practice interacting with like-minded peers and become familiar with what research involves. Participation in scientific competitions is a good way to stand out when applying to medical schools or doctoral programs.

Talk to professionals in the field. You can find both neurologists and researchers at teaching hospitals and universities. Simply call one of these institutions and ask to speak to someone in the neurology department. Try to arrange to job shadow several different kinds of neurology professionals to get an idea of what area would best suit you. Most professors and researchers will be happy to show you around and talk to you about what the work entails.

Bolster your college application by volunteering at a hospital or similar medical environment. Another way to gain valuable hands-on experience is to get a part-time job in healthcare. It does not have to be in neurology to be useful. Any healthcare job will help you determine if a career in medicine would be a good fit.

Join professional associations such as the American Neurological Association, Society for Neuroscience, or Association of Clinical Research Professionals. These are national associations, but there are also many regional organizations. Check to see if there are any in your area so you can easily attend workshops and seminars.

HISTORY OF THE CAREERS

NEUROSCIENCE IS A RELATIVELY NEW scientific discipline, with most modern methods having been developed in the mid-20th century. However, the mysteries of the brain have been a source of fascination since the earliest of times. In fact, a form of brain surgery has been around since the Stone Age. Trepanation is a surgical procedure in which a hole is drilled or scraped into the human skull to relieve pressure or expose the dura mater for treatment of health problems. Evidence collected from skeletal remains revealed that the Incas used trepanation to treat injured warriors – though evidence also shows that the results were usually fatal. Still, the procedure was continued and improved, and it is not that different from brain surgery performed today.

The ancient Egyptians were the first to write about the brain, around 3000 BC. The Edwin Smith Papyrus, circa 1700 BC, is the earliest existing medical text. It included discussions of the brain, the meninges, the spinal cord, and cerebrospinal fluid. Seven medical cases involving treating traumatic brain injuries were also described.

The ancient Greeks also studied the nervous system. Physician Hippocrates declared that epilepsy had a natural cause, rejecting the traditional religious connections. Aristotle described the meninges, cerebrum, and cerebellum, and Plato determined that mental processes originated in the brain, not the heart.

In the Middle Ages, Roman physician Galen performed many experiments on the nervous system to investigate what causes mental health disorders. His findings made a significant contribution to the knowledge of human anatomy in general and neuroscience in particular. Galen believed that the brain controlled bodily functions as well as a person's temperament, a radically new theory at that time.

The Renaissance

In 1543 the first true medical textbook to include neuroscience was published by Flemish physician, Andreas Vesalius. *On the Fabric of the Human Body* was a seven-volume set of books that was considered revolutionary. It included detailed images of cranial nerves, meninges, ventricles, the peripheral nerves, and the vascular supply to the brain and spinal cord. The text was followed a few years later by the first book devoted to neurology, *De Cerebri Morbis*. In this text, Dutch physician Jason Pratensis, discussed specific symptoms of neurological diseases and theorized on their origins.

Advances continued in the mid-17th century, with Thomas Willis' books, *Anatomy of the Brain* and *Cerebral*

Pathology. Willis was the first to remove the brain from the cranium for purposes of scientific study. He was able to prove some of his ideas about brain functions and described epilepsy, apoplexy, and paralysis in his books. Willis was also the first to use the word "neurology."

The Neurology Specialty Is Established

The 19th century saw the first physicians to devote their practice entirely to neurology. The development of specialized tools and procedures spurred the advance of the specialty throughout the century. Some of the most significant tools were the tendon hammer, ophthalmoscope, syringe, and lumbar puncture. Using the "modern" techniques, Scottish surgeon, William McEwen, was able to perform the first successful neurosurgery to remove a brain tumor In 1878. Three years later, Victor Horsley was able to remove a spinal tumor.

By the end of the century, the cause and effect of numerous neurological conditions had been established, including stroke and hemiplegia, trauma and paraplegia, spirochaete (a type of bacteria), and paralytic dementia. One of the pioneering neurologists, Paul Broca, discovered the part of the brain that produced speech. Neuroscientists also began to compare their findings with those of a new kind of scientist, the neuropathologist.

20th Century

We have come a long way since ancient Egypt. Most of what neurologists are now able to do evolved from developments in the 20th century. Hans Berger invented the electroencephalography (EEG), a device that measures electrical activity in the brain, in 1929. Electrodes were discovered in the 19th century, but it was not until 1950 that Dr. Jose Delgado was able to implant an electrode in an animal's brain and use it to control the animal's movements.

In 1928, Isidor Rabi discovered nuclear magnetic resonance, the foundation of magnetic resonance imaging (MRI). This was a turning point for neuroscience. Before the development of MRI machines, the brain was shrouded in mystery, but with an MRI, neurologists could see what was happening inside. In 1992, fMRI (functional MRI) was first used to map activity in the human brain.

The cochlear implant, a neurological prosthetic that allows deaf people to hear, was introduced to the public in 1972. Neuroscience researcher, Philip Kennedy, implanted the first Brain Computer Interface (BCI) into a human subject. Numerous technological developments further enhanced the field, such as the Positron Emission Tomography (PET) scanner and CAT scans.

Today, neuroscience is still a fledgling discipline and there is much more to be learned. Neuroscientists are hard at work, mapping the vast human nervous system. In 2009, the National Institutes of Health (NIH) sponsored the launch of the Human Connectome Project. The goal is to produce a highly detailed map of the human nervous system with its millions of connections. This kind of neural mapping is expected to lead to the diagnosis and treatment of many neurological disorders that are today considered untreatable.

WHERE YOU WILL WORK

MOST NEUROSCIENTISTS WORK IN AN ACADEMIC environment. Upon finishing their doctoral programs, almost 40 percent continue with research, and the others become faculty members. Together these groups spend the majority of their time conducting research funded by their academic institutions, the government, or medical research organizations. A small percentage of time is spent in the classroom teaching the next generation of neuroscientists. Only one in five proceed directly to jobs outside of academia. Most of their employers are research and development firms, medical and diagnostic laboratories, and hospitals. Some work for the federal government.

Currently, there are about 16,000 neurologists employed in the US. Unlike other types of physicians and surgeons, these professionals rarely maintain their own private offices due to the nature of the work. Instead, they are likely to be employed by hospitals, healthcare organizations, or the government. Some do work in group practices where they share a large number of patients with doctors of other specialties that complement neurology. The group setting is less stressful than the hospital because there is more freedom to control the flow of patients and take time off when needed.

Work Environment

Like all scientists, neuroscientists spend most of their working hours in laboratories and offices, studying data and reports. The workstations are clean, well lit, and are outfitted with the most modern equipment. Occasionally, the work involves dangerous biological samples and chemicals, but neuroscientists are trained to take proper safety precautions, so accidents are rare.

The typical work environment of a neurologist depends on the type of condition the doctor specializes in. For example, a neurologist specializing in inherited neurological diseases might split the time between seeing patients and conducting research. Their patients often provide the basis for their studies. A neurologist specializing in head traumas might work in an emergency healthcare setting, and provide follow-up care in the primary care unit of the hospital. A neurosurgeon would work in a sterile environment while performing surgery and may also have an office located in the hospital.

Both neuroscientists and neurologists work full time, and the hours tend to be fairly regular. However, in the hospital environment it is not unusual for neurologists to be on call to deal with neurological problems that may arise in emergency rooms at any time of the day or night. Normally, there is not much travel involved in this work, but being on call does present situations that may require an emergency visit to a hospital or nursing home.

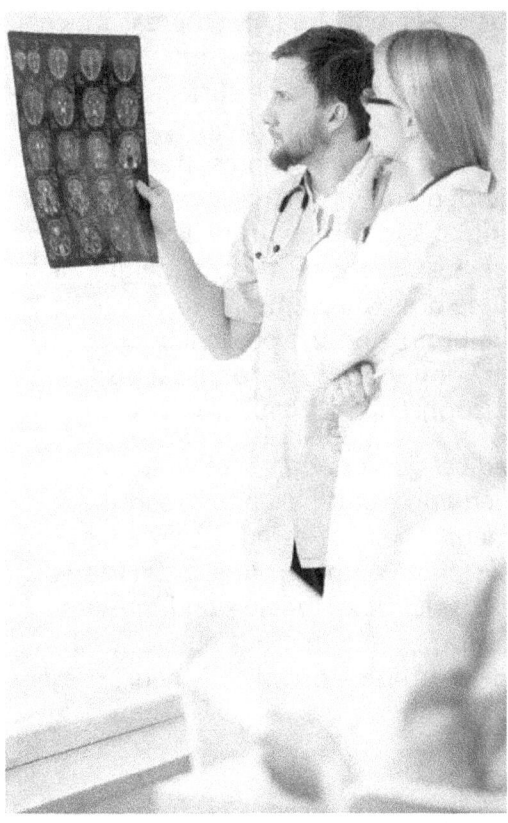

THE WORK YOU WILL DO

NEUROSCIENCE IS THE STUDY OF THE NERVOUS SYSTEM, its structure, how it develops, and what it does. It is a sweeping field that covers many areas from psychology to genetics to computer science. Neuroscientists are interested in how the nervous system develops, its structure, and what it does. They primarily focus on the brain and how it impacts behavior and cognitive functions, but the nervous system goes well beyond the brain, encompassing the spinal cord and nerve cells throughout the body.

The field of neuroscience is in its infancy. There is much to be learned about the nervous system and neuroscientists have only scratched the surface. Cutting edge research is continually probing the workings of the human mind and its effects on all systems of the body. Some call this the golden age of neuroscience because research is developing at such a rapid rate. Each new discovery – and there are dozens that come to light each year – leads to genuine breakthroughs in our understanding of the brain, and the possibility of overcoming previously intractable neurological disorders like Alzheimer's, schizophrenia, and autism.

Neurologists are medical doctors that take what neuro-scientists have learned and put it into practice in the healthcare environment. Their concern is disorders of the brain and nervous system. Neurological disorders can also include diseases that affect blood vessels and muscles. Neurology is a medical specialty that has numerous subspecialties, the most notable of which is neurosurgery.

What Neuroscientists Do

Neuroscientists spend most of their time researching the origins of neurological problems. Some projects are experimental and are seen as "pure research" to advance the knowledge base in the field. Other projects are specifically intended to formulate cures or treatments. Pharmaceutical firms, for example, are eager to develop new medicine or other biotechnology products for the millions of consumers now suffering from neurological disorders.

Most of the neuroscientist's work takes place in laboratories at private research centers, government facilities, and universities. Unlike neurologists, neuroscientists involved in research do not work directly with patients, although patients may be subjects of test cases. There are exceptions, however. Neuroscientists may also be licensed neurologists and neurosurgeons who treat patients.

Specific tasks vary depending on the scope of the research project. It could be anything from developing new medical equipment or methodology for analyzing data, to determining whether there are genetic links to certain psychiatric disorders or what happens to an aging brain. Some neuroscientists specialize in a specific part of the nervous system such as neurotransmitters, while others focus on certain illnesses such as Parkinson's.

Most research projects start with collecting and preparing tissue and cell samples. Dyes, antibodies, and gene probes are used to identify different components. Brain and nerve activity is monitored with various kinds of medical tools and imaging equipment. Microelectrodes attached to the head combined with magnetic resonance imagers (MRI) make it possible for a neuroscientist to watch the brain at work. Computers are central to all research projects. They are used for everything from collecting and analyzing data to creating entire nervous system models.

When potential new treatments are discovered, they need to be tested. Tests conducted on mice or monkeys can indicate how the medication would affect the human brain. Animal testing can take a long time to understand how a drug interacts with brain processes and determine if there are any side effects. Only after the drug is found to be safe as well as effective does it start the clinical trial phase, which involves human subjects.

Neurology

Neurology is a medical specialty that involves treating health problems that are caused by and/or affect the nervous system. Problems like migraines, epilepsy, brain tumors, and traumatic head injuries are obviously directly related to the brain. However, neurological problems can have a negative impact on the functioning of any body part or system because the brain is the central command of the entire human body. Problems may show up as tremors, loss of muscle function, seizures, sleep disorders, lack of sensitivity to pain or temperature, eyesight impairment, or inability to swallow or speak.

Because the nervous system affects every part of the body, neurologists may be flooded with a vast array of patients seeking treatment. There are more than 1 billion people worldwide who suffer from neurological disorders – that is one out of six people! Many cannot be treated and some will die. Some of the most common problems are progressive diseases such as Huntington's and Lou Gehrig's disease. Others, like multiple sclerosis, are caused by damage to nerve cells. There are traumatic injuries to the brain or spinal cord. There are chronic conditions like diabetes or vasculitis that cause painful peripheral nerve damage.

Depending on the situation, a neurologist may need to provide acute care to patients who are suddenly afflicted by a serious problem. In the case of chronic conditions like Alzheimer's or Parkinson's, the neurologist may become the patient's principal care physician.

An overlap between neurology and psychiatry is common. Some mental illnesses are classified as psychiatric diseases, yet the root of the problem is a neurological disorder. For example, a neurochemical imbalance is believed to be behind schizophrenia and bipolar disorder, two conditions considered mental illness.

What Neurologists Do

Every neurology case begins with a diagnosis. This can be a daunting task since the nervous system is so extensive and so little understood. The neurologist first needs to pinpoint the origin of the symptoms. This is done through a neurological exam, which usually involves cranial nerve tests, mental status tests, and evaluations of reflexes, sensation, coordination, and strength. During the initial examination, the neurologist will review the patient's health history and try to connect past issues with the current condition.

In some cases, more sophisticated diagnostic tests are needed. Advanced imaging tools such as Computer Tomography (CT), Magnetic Resonance Imaging (MRI), and ultrasound of major blood vessels in the head and neck are invaluable for providing visual details. Other common tests include neurophysiologic studies such as electroencephalography (EEG), needle electromyography (EMG), nerve conduction studies (NCSs), and Evoked Potential (EP) tests that measure the electrical activity of the brain in response to stimulation of sensory nerve pathways. Neurologists also perform lumbar punctures to assess a patient's cerebrospinal fluid.

An exciting new area of diagnostics is genetic testing. Recent advances in this area have made it a vital tool in the classification of inherited neuromuscular diseases and diagnosis of many other neurogenetic diseases.

Only after an accurate diagnosis has been reached can treatment begin. This could mean prescribing medications, recommending a surgical procedure, or referral to a specialist such as a physiotherapist, speech pathologist, or psychiatrist. In some cases, there is no effective treatment yet available. In other cases, there may be a way to manage the condition even though there is no cure.

What a Neurosurgeon Does

When treatment requires surgery, the neurologist will refer the case to a neurosurgeon. A neurosurgeon is a specialist who has spent additional years of medical training to perform the most delicate operations on the brain and spinal cord. After a surgery, the patient is usually back in the care of the neurologist for long-term follow up.

Both neurologists and neurosurgeons can choose to specialize in a specific area of practice. Common subspecialties include pediatric, geriatric, spinal cord injuries, and behavioral disorders, but this is an expansive field with many more subspecialties to choose from. Neurologists can focus on particular parts of the nervous system such as peripheral nerve fibers, while others only perform specific procedures like diagnostic studies. Subspecialties can also be devoted to particular disorders, especially common ones like epilepsy, sleep disorders, autism, or dementia.

Since neurological issues overlap with many other disciplines, there are numerous associated specialties, including genetic counseling, speech language pathology, and cognitive neuroscience.

STORIES OF PROFESSIONALS IN THE FIELD

I Work in a Teaching Hospital

"The neurosurgeons on TV are exciting heroes, but the reality is anything but glamorous. The work is truly rewarding, but it's also very hard work. My day starts before sunrise with patient rounds, reviewing research, supervising residents, and managing staff. Throughout the day, there are the inevitable mad dashes to the ER to treat car crash victims with traumatic head injuries. And after the sun goes down, I'm still at it, catching up on dictation.

The worst part of this job is breaking bad news to heartbroken loved ones. People expect us to be gods who can cure anything, but there are many neurological problems that can't be fixed. Yet that is what pushes me to stay involved in research projects. Every little bit of new information is another piece in the puzzle that will someday save many more lives or make life more enjoyable for millions. What if my late night experiments result in a breakthrough that leads to the ability to reverse the prenatal brain damage? That would mean more than 700,000 kids could be spared the ravages of Cerebral Palsy. Just knowing I'm contributing to that possible outcome makes all the endless days and hard work worth it."

I Am a Neurosurgeon

"I specialize in brain trauma. I handle the most severe emergencies on very short notice and make life-or-death decisions every day. Most cases are the result of car accidents or older people falling. Having someone's brain health in my hands is both exhilarating and humbling because I know that in a split second, things can go wrong. I never let fear affect my confidence because I know the odds are about 10 to one that my skills will produce a good outcome.

Med students should take the time to carefully consider their specialty before committing. What excites you more, doing cutting-edge research or operating on human brains? Fewer hospitals are allowing neurosurgeons to do both because of the demands on time. If you say surgery is your passion, then try a bunch of different subspecialties during residency. I tried spine surgery, pediatric neurosurgery, and cerebrovascular surgery before deciding neurotrauma was where I belonged.

You must also be determined to take excellent care of yourself. The work is exhausting and there is little time for working out or eating a nutritious meal, but you have to do it if you're going to be at your best during surgery. I get to bed early, make time for a good breakfast, go for runs during lunch, and drink tons of water. You absolutely cannot be sleep-deprived, hungry, or dehydrated when somebody's life is in your hands.

Despite all the challenges, I can't imagine a more satisfying job. The gratitude in a family member's eyes when a surgery goes well and you can tell them their loved one will be fine is not something you can find in the typical job."

I Treat Neuromuscular Diseases

"My patients come to the clinic with all kinds of neuropathies, from headaches and tingling toes to multiple sclerosis and Parkinson's disease. My day is a mix of doing diagnostic procedures like electromyography and muscle biopsies, to treating patients with immunosuppressive drugs and Botox injections. Many neurological conditions are chronic, meaning there is no cure, but most can be managed. What makes my work so interesting is the ever-growing array of treatment options. Right now, there are more than a dozen different treatment options for multiple sclerosis alone!

I also teach medical students and residents completing their training in the clinic, and occasionally give guest lectures. I wish I could do more teaching because there is a critical shortage of neurologists. I'd like to help bridge the gap, but that same shortage keeps me too busy to add any more teaching duties to my schedule. Instead, I tell anyone who will listen that neurology is a rapidly growing field with tons of exciting options and opportunities."

PERSONAL QUALIFICATIONS

NEUROLOGY PROFESSIONALS ARE FOCUSED individuals who are passionate about their work, have the intellect to understand the complexities of the field, and are good at making critical decisions without hesitation. The most successful people in this career share a number of other innate skills that help them with their day-to-day tasks.

Communication Skills

Communication skills are critical in all areas of neurology. Neurologists must be able to gather information and assess situations quickly. Patients can be any age and will come from all walks of life. Being able to talk to everyone in terms they can understand is a big plus. Since patients with neurological disorders often experience some type of deficit in cognition, motor skills, or speech, patience and compassion are needed. As specialists, neurologists collaborate extensively with other healthcare providers, making strong communication skills on a professional level very important.

Communication is also critical in research in order to explain project goals and conclusions. Writing is a particularly important skill for neuroscientists. These professionals may spend considerable time writing grant proposals, which are needed to fund their research. Neurology professionals are also expected to be published in medical journals. A good reputation is often the result of a well-written article.

Critical Thinking Skills

Those going into the research end of neuroscience should possess a high level of intellectual curiosity and an academic attitude. Neurology professionals spend at least 12 years in school mastering the necessary factual knowledge to work in the field. They must also possess the ability to access and analyze relevant data to determine the best solution for specific research questions. This requires a balance of technical proficiency and creativity.

Observation Skills

Whether working with patients or on a project in a laboratory, neurology requires precise observation of data, samples, and behavior. In this field, the tiniest detail can have an enormous impact. There is no room for sloppiness when mistakes can have deadly consequences. A successful neurology professional has the unique ability to focus on every detail while grasping a broad understanding of the bigger picture.

Teamwork

Neurology professionals must be equally comfortable working alone as well as being a team member. In the clinical setting neurologists rely on a number of other medical professionals. Teamwork is essential in the lab, too, where cooperation is key. Different members on the lab team will have different responsibilities. For example, one person may prepare samples while another assists graduate students. After an experiment is set up, others will collect and analyze the data. At the end of the experiment, all members of the team are expected to participate in discussions and brainstorm to figure out what the next steps should be.

Leadership

In the research environment, success of a lab often depends on the leadership skills of the neuroscientists. Research is surprisingly competitive and every lab is vying to attract the best graduate students and post-doctoral fellows to work on their projects. A good leader understands that different people have different skills and is able to match the right people to the right projects. Leadership also involves motivating people. A successful neuroscientist knows how to get people to work more efficiently, as well as when to push or when to encourage with praise.

ATTRACTIVE FEATURES

NEUROLOGY IS A FASCINATING FIELD. The human brain and the nervous system are considered the final frontier of medical science. Little is known about how the neurological system affects all other aspects of the human condition, making it a wide-open field for research far into the future. Those who love science will find the work especially intellectually satisfying. It is very challenging work, but it often involves some of the most interesting cases in medicine.

The work offers many professional and personal rewards. Neurological disorders are often complex with vague symptoms that most doctors overlook or misunderstand. Patients with these disorders sometimes go undiagnosed for months, and after going through countless tests, they are left feeling discouraged and helpless. When a neurologist is able to provide answers, it is a tremendous relief for the patient and the family. Imagine being called in on a tough case that stumps the entire healthcare team, and after just talking to and examining the patient, you are able to pinpoint the problem. It is an amazing feeling. For the neuroscientist who spends every day seeking to unlock the mysteries of the brain, the prize is a discovery that will help millions of people live healthier, happier lives.

In this day of specialization, there are many kinds of doctors, yet neurologists may be the most highly respected. They are considered the "doctor's doctor," with unmatched expertise in their field. Other doctors and healthcare professionals consult them on the most complex cases. It is not by accident "brain surgeon" is a cliché that describes the smartest among us. One can only imagine the ego boost that comes from penetrating a person's skull and performing brain surgery.

Most choose this career for the love of the work. Neurology professionals are passionate about medical science and enjoy the opportunity to contribute to the body of knowledge about the nervous system. While their satisfaction cannot be measured in dollars and cents, they are very well compensated. Depending on where they work, neurologists typically enjoy the highest earnings among all doctors. For example, a neurosurgeon in New York City can expect to earn more than half a million dollars a year! Likewise, neuroscientists who conduct their research on behalf of pharmaceutical companies are among the highest paid scientists. Their earnings typically top $100,000 annually.

Neurology offers unparalleled opportunities with a job growth rate that is much faster than that of other occupations. Due to the severe shortage of qualified neurologists, anyone considering the challenge of 12 years of training can be assured there will be a job waiting. There is competition for the many neuroscience graduates who plan on a career in academia, but there is also job stability for most. A neuroscientist with tenure at a university essentially has a job for life. Those who do not attain tenure are less secure, with their future being dependent on obtaining grants to continue their work.

UNATTRACTIVE ASPECTS

THE MAIN DISADVANTAGE TO A CAREER in neurology is the high barrier to entry. Educational requirements are lengthy and intense. It takes about 12 years to earn a PhD or MD and attain the relevant license to practice. That takes a high level of commitment, dedication, and patience – the same attributes needed to practice in the field once a career is launched. This kind of education is also expensive. Fortunately, there should be an excellent salary available to help pay off student loans after graduation.

Neurologists can experience stress. They often work on difficult cases that require long hours. In some cases, a neurosurgeon's success will make the difference between life and death. There is a high rate of burnout in neurology. The American Academy of Neurology (AAN) reports that more than half the organization's members experience at least one symptom of burnout or emotional exhaustion. This problem is exacerbated by the shortage of neurologists, which necessitates patient overload that tends to lead to work-life imbalance.

Neurologists are trained to dig through obscure clues to reach a correct conclusion. Some cases are difficult to diagnose, especially when there are more patients than hours in the day. Because of the shortage of neurologists, there is increasing pressure to see too many patients and cut the time spent with each. Neurologists take pride in solving neurological problems, and patients want answers, but diagnosis and treatment are not always possible. Neurology is still in its infancy, and there are many neurological disorders that have no effective treatment. It can be difficult explaining to people that medical science is not as advanced as they would like it to be.

Instant gratification is rarely seen in this field. Neurology professionals of all kinds need endless patience. Research projects can take years to produce clear conclusions. Similarly, patient progress can be slow. Even with proper treatment, neurological disorders may improve only a little over time.

EDUCATION AND TRAINING

THE EDUCATIONAL REQUIREMENTS are different for neurologists and neuroscientists. Neurologists are medical doctors who must earn an MD by attending medical school and completing a residency. Neurosurgeons spend additional time studying general and specialized surgical procedures. Depending on the subspecialty, it can take anywhere from 8 to 15 years to become a practicing neurologist.

Neuroscientists generally earn a PhD degree. It is possible to get into the field of neuroscience with only a bachelor's degree. That would qualify you for a paying job as a research assistant in most private research facilities and university laboratories. Assistants can perform many of the tasks involved in research projects, but there is a limit to how far they can advance, and the pay will never come close to that of a neuroscientist with a PhD. Moving into higher positions usually requires at least a master's degree where extensive classroom and laboratory work are focused on a specific area of neurology research.

Undergraduate Work

Becoming a neurologist starts with earning a bachelor's degree. Technically, an undergraduate can major in any field, but there is an obvious advantage to focusing on biological sciences, chemistry, or physics. There are also admission requirements for medical school to be considered. Pre-med requisite courses typically include microbiology, organic chemistry, and human anatomy.

To be eligible for medical school, third year undergraduates must take and pass the Medical College Admission Test (MCAT). The purpose of the exam is to evaluate an applicant's training and knowledge, and allow medical schools to determine whether the student is prepared for the rigors of medical school.

Aspiring neuroscientists usually major in neuroscience or one of the other main biological sciences. Chemistry or psychology majors are also common. Coursework includes a broad range of subjects, including life sciences, physics, computer science, cognitive science, and advanced mathematics. There are usually several statistics and laboratory courses where you learn about research techniques, laboratory equipment, and data manipulation. Instruction in how to write scientific papers is provided though students are advised to take additional communication classes that will help them write compelling grants and get research findings published.

Undergraduates may gain field experience by working as an intern or assistant in a university research program. Most schools require students to conduct independent research and write a dissertation to obtain their degrees.

Graduate Studies

Graduate programs for neuroscientists allow students to focus on particular areas such as neurobiology, cognitive neuroscience, or pharmacology. Classroom instruction is directed entirely on neuroscience topics like neural circuitry, proteomics, and cognitive and behavioral pathologies. Graduate students spend the bulk of their time in the laboratory environment, learning processes and techniques such as microarray analysis, gene splicing, and brain imaging. At this level, students are expected to develop their own original research projects and eventually supervise undergraduates.

Neuroscientists who want to devote their careers to research are not required to have medical training, but it is advantageous. Only licensed physicians can administer drugs and therapies to human patients in clinical trials. Some schools offer dual-degree programs that combine a PhD with a neurology medical degree. A typical neuroscience PhD program is focused on research methods, such as project design and data interpretation. Students in dual-degree programs learn those same research skills, but are also trained in the clinical skills needed to be a physician.

Graduate students planning careers in neurology need to attend medical school and earn a Doctor of Medicine degree (MD). It usually takes four years to complete medical school. The first two years include instruction in general medical subjects such as physiology, human anatomy, pharmacology, pathology, immunology, biochemistry, and medical law. Training also covers how to examine patients, record medical histories, and diagnose health problems. During the last two years, med students can opt for specific clinical training in neurology. Training is provided in both classroom and laboratory settings throughout the four years.

Residency

After medical school, neurologists move into a three-year neurology residency program accredited by the Accreditation Council for Graduate Medical Education. During this time, they continue to attend required lectures, participate in patient rounds, and complete case studies of a variety of neurological disorders and procedures, such as dementia, epilepsy, and neuroradiology.

Fellowships

Not all students participate in fellowship programs, but those who do gain detailed knowledge of specialized areas of neurology from experienced faculty and medical teams. Fellowships at university medical facilities or teaching hospitals generally last one or two years.

Aspiring neuroscientists may also find fellowships with research institutions. Fellows in this type of program would work alongside experienced scientists to gain a detailed understanding of neurology research. They would be expected to perform all the normal tasks of a researcher, including writing grant proposals, facilitating clinical trials, and publishing scientific papers. The fellowship may last more than two years, after which there would be an opportunity to begin conducting independent research.

Licensing and Certifications

Neuroscientists who primarily conduct research do not need licenses or certifications. However, in order to treat patients, neuroscientists must earn an MD degree, participate in a medical residency, and pass the United States Medical Licensing Examination. There are also voluntary certifications for qualified neurologists offered by the American Board of Psychology and Neurology (ABPN).

EARNINGS

THE AVERAGE ANNUAL SALARY OF medical scientists working at pharmaceutical and other medicine manufacturing companies is about $110,000. The comparable figure for medical scientists employed by colleges and universities is about $75,000.

The median annual salary earned by all neuroscientists depends on the type of employer and what the work involves. The median annual salary is around $80,000, but those working for pharmaceutical or other medicine manufacturing companies can earn considerably more – just over $100,000. Research and development firms pay slightly less. Although most neuroscientists seek jobs in academia, that is where earnings are the lowest. However, this employment also offers the greatest potential job security and most opportunities to work on cutting-edge research projects. Only a small number of neuroscientists earn less than $50,000 a year.

Neurologist salaries also vary greatly by specialty, location, and years of experience. Median earnings are about $190,000, but there is a huge range - from $150,000 to $300,000. With the right combination of location, reputation, and specialty, earnings can be very high. For example, a neurosurgeon in a major hospital in New York City could earn $600,000 a year. Outside of New York, the highest paying state for neurologists is Florida, where the median annual income is $375,000. The reason for Florida's high ranking is likely due to the population that has a higher percentage of older adults than other states. This has caused a severe shortage of neurologists to serve aging Baby Boomers and other retirees who experience increased rates of age-related neurological disorders like Alzheimer's.

OPPORTUNITIES

ALTHOUGH NEUROSCIENCE AND NEUROLOGY are closely associated, there are considerable differences in the job outlook for each.

The job growth rate for neuroscience is expected to be roughly eight percent over the coming decade. That is about average when compared to other professions. On the plus side, there are several factors that will contribute to more opportunities for neuroscientists. The aging population will continue to grow along with increased rates of several age-related chronic conditions, such as Alzheimer's. There is an urgent need for researchers to find treatments for such conditions now considered incurable. Alzheimer's alone affects 7 million older Americans and more than 44 million people worldwide.

Each new discovery in medical science provides a greater understanding of the nervous system processes, but a discovery is never an end in itself. Instead, it leads neuroscientists into new areas of research. In addition, our dependence on pharmaceutical treatments will continue to grow as fast as researchers can create them.

It is understood that the work of neuroscientists contributes to the overall improvement of human health. Therefore, the government will continue to be a major source of funding for neuroscientific research. Going forward, the majority of research grants will be funded at the federal level.

While many new opportunities for neuroscientists will continue to open up, there is no shortage of qualified candidates to fill the jobs. It is an exciting field that has attracted many dedicated scientists. Interest in the field will continue to drive the number of new graduates with PhDs to take those positions.

While there may be an adequate number of neuro-scientists, the opposite is true of neurologists, who are doctors with MD degrees. In fact, there is a severe shortage that is not predicted to peak until well into the future. The pace of job growth is accelerating at a rate much faster than that of other occupations. There will be an estimated 18,000 practicing neurologists, but that is not enough to keep up with the growth trend, which will be 20 percent over the next decade. Government projections as well as independent studies predict that there will be over 21,000 job openings, a shortfall of at least 3,000 of these doctors.

The shortage is good news for new graduates, as almost all will have their residencies lined up before they even finish medical school. The intense demand for neurology services is primarily driven by the same factor as neuroscience – an aging population. Alzheimer's, Parkinson's disease, and stroke are on the rise, and Baby Boomers are starting to experience various forms of dementia. Greater numbers than ever before will seek high levels of care that employ the latest technologies, diagnostic tests, and therapies. The demand continues to grow, far outpacing the supply of these professionals.

Those who are willing to practice in rural and low-income areas will find particularly good prospects since these areas usually have difficulty attracting all kinds of physicians. While the shortage of neurologists affects the entire country, the situation is worse in certain locations. The Alzheimer's Association reported recently that there are multiple regions of the US that will see a rapid rise in

Alzheimer's and other types of dementia. These areas, which will experience a chronic shortage of neurologists, are described as neurology "deserts."

Neurocern is a computer program that analyzes symptoms in order to provide diagnostic guidance for doctors and a personalized care plan for patients. Using data from the Centers for Medicare and Medicaid Services, they have developed the Alzheimer's Disease and Related Disorders Neurology Desert Index (ANDI). The data reveal a great imbalance between states in terms of available services. Twenty states are identified as dementia neurology "deserts" with the most significant disparity in Wyoming, North Dakota, South Carolina, South Dakota, and Oklahoma.

GETTING STARTED

THERE IS MUCH YOU CAN DO TO PREPARE for a successful career launch while still in college. There are numerous choices in specialties, working settings, and ways to apply your knowledge and skills. Are you interested in studying behavioral disorders or has DNA sequencing got you fascinated? Do you want to work with children, older adults, or just anybody who could use your expertise? Would you rather work in a well-equipped laboratory or a surgical suite? Whether you want to work in research, academia, clinical medicine, or industry, you need to carefully investigate your options and steer your efforts in the direction of your choice.

You will likely be offered at least one class in grant writing. Future neuroscientists should take advantage of this opportunity. One of the most effective ways to get noticed as a neuroscientist is to become an expert grant writer. Every research project is dependent on securing funding from health and science organizations. Offer to help your professors draft grant proposals. If one is successful, it will be a huge plus on your résumé. For extra practice, you can get a part-time job writing grant proposals. It will be time well spent and you will be well paid.

Start joining professional associations while you are a student. It is a good way to stay up to date with the latest technology in the field. It is also an excellent source of potential job connections. Professional associations like the Society for Neuroscience offer workshops, seminars, conferences, and other resources for members. Most associations also maintain job boards and advertise openings in their journals.

Get as much hands-on experience as you can. Internships will be a vital part of your training. In some cases, a successful internship will eventually lead to a full-time job offer.

Look for opportunities to volunteer at community service organizations, community health centers, and nursing homes. These places always need extra help and in return, you will make valuable contacts.

  Start looking for a mentor right away. You need someone who can give advice, guide you toward your career goals, and provide recommendations during your first job search. Faculty members are often willing to be mentors. Another possibility is the senior researcher who supervises your doctoral studies.

The value of networking cannot be underestimated in this field. Start building connections early by talking to your professors during office hours. Ask which seminars, workshops, conferences, and other industry events you should attend. Showing up is a good start, but you should also make an effort to interact with established professionals and seek out those who specialize in the areas that interest you. Take advantage of the question and answer sessions that typically follow most events. You can clarify issues you might have, and you can demonstrate to potential contacts your dedication to the field.

While networking is the primary source of job leads, there are other ways to get started. Your college placement center will have listings of job openings. Check with your department head, too. It is common for research centers and hospitals to have relationships with faculty members. Post your résumé on professional association job boards and check their journals for advertised jobs. You can also use employment agencies that specialize in medical and scientific research careers.

Most neurologists have their first jobs lined up by the time they complete their residency or fellowship. For the few that do not, or for those who are undecided on which specialty to pursue, neurology locum tenens positions may be the perfect solution. Locum tenens positions are temporary contract jobs that vary in position, setting, location, and compensation. Generally, the pay is very good, the duration averages six months, and the location can be just about anywhere you choose.

ASSOCIATIONS

■ **Society for Neuroscience**
http://www.sfn.org

■ **Association of Clinical Research Professionals**
https://www.acrpnet.org

■ **American Neurological Association**
https://myana.org

■ **American Academy of Neurology**
https://www.aan.com

PERIODICALS

■ **Journal of Neurological Sciences**
http://www.jns-journal.com

■ **Pediatric Neurology**
http://www.pedneur.com

■ **Brain and Development**
http://www.brainanddevelopment.com

■ **Journal of Neurology**
http://www.neurology.org

WEBSITE

■ **Neurocern**
https://www.neurocern.com